Copyright © 2023 By Lisa Madison

All Right Reserved.

This document is geared towards providing exact and reliable information in regards to the topic and issue covered. The publication is sold with the idea that the publisher is not required to render an account officially permitted or otherwise qualified services. If advice is necessary, legal or professional, a practiced individual in the profession should be ordered.

In no way is it legal to reproduce, duplicate, or transmit any part of this document by either electronic means or in printed format. The recording of this publication is strictly prohibited, and any storage of this document is not allowed unless with written permission from the publisher. All rights reserved.

The information provided herein is stated to be truthful and consistent. In terms of inattention or otherwise, any liability, by any use or abuse of any policies, processes, or directions contained within is the solitary and utter responsibility of the recipient reader. Under no circumstances will any reparation, damages, or monetary indirectly

Disclaimer Notice: Please note the information contained within this document is for educational and entertainment purposes only. Every attempt has been made to provide accurate, up to date and reliable, complete information. No warranties of any kind are expressed or implied. Reader acknowledges that the author is not engaging in the rendering of legal, financial, medical, or professional advice. The content of this book has been derived from various sources. Please consult a licensed professional before attempting any techniques outlined in this book.

TABLE OF CONTENTS

Wall Pilates Workouts	04
INTRODUCTION	08
WALL PILATES BENEFITS	11
28-DAYS CALLENGE	17
DAYS 1-5	18
DAYS 6-10	28
DAYS 11-15	39
DAYS 16-20	50
DAYS 21-25	61
DAYS 26-28	72
CONCLUSION	79

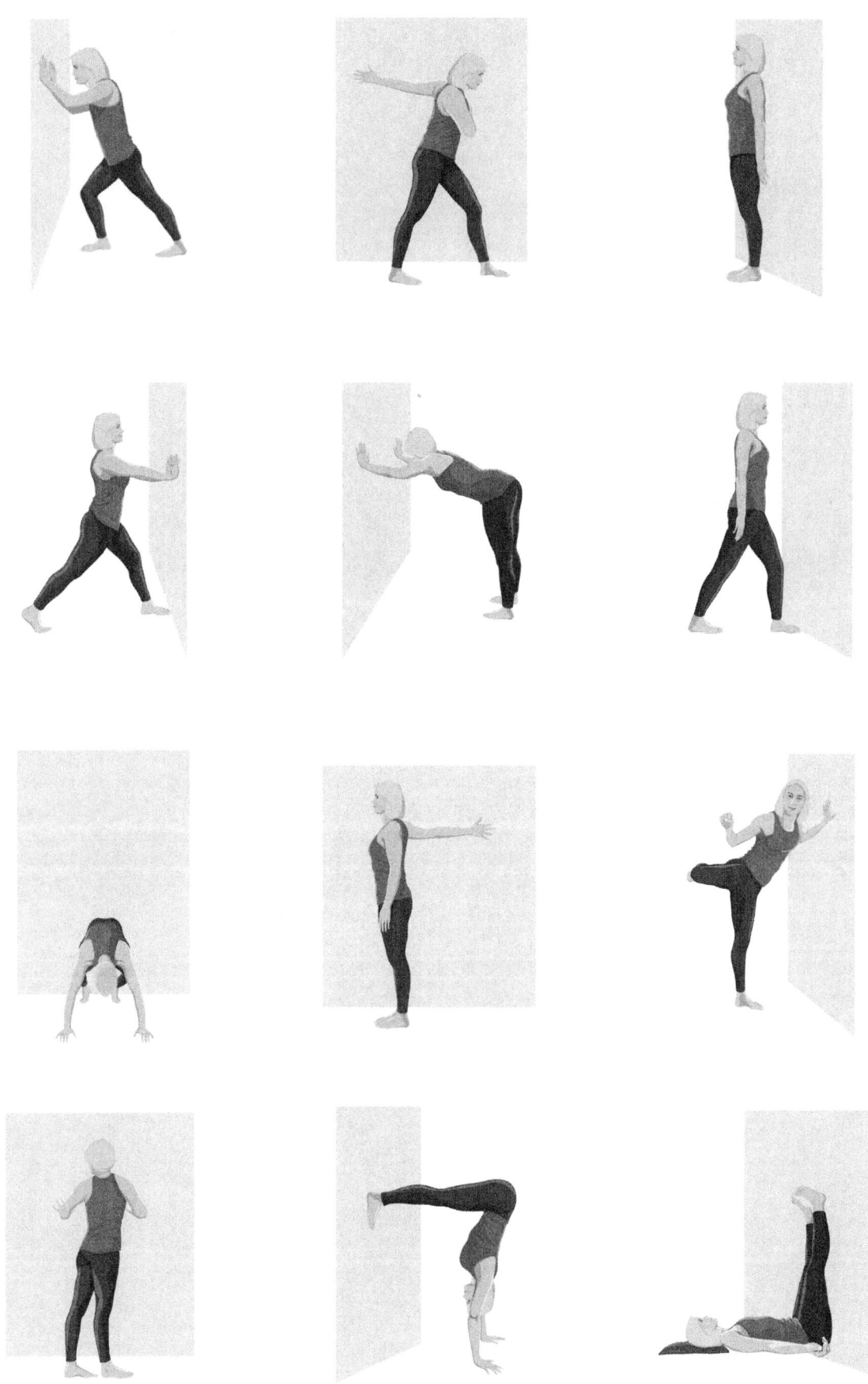

WALL PILATES WORKOUTS

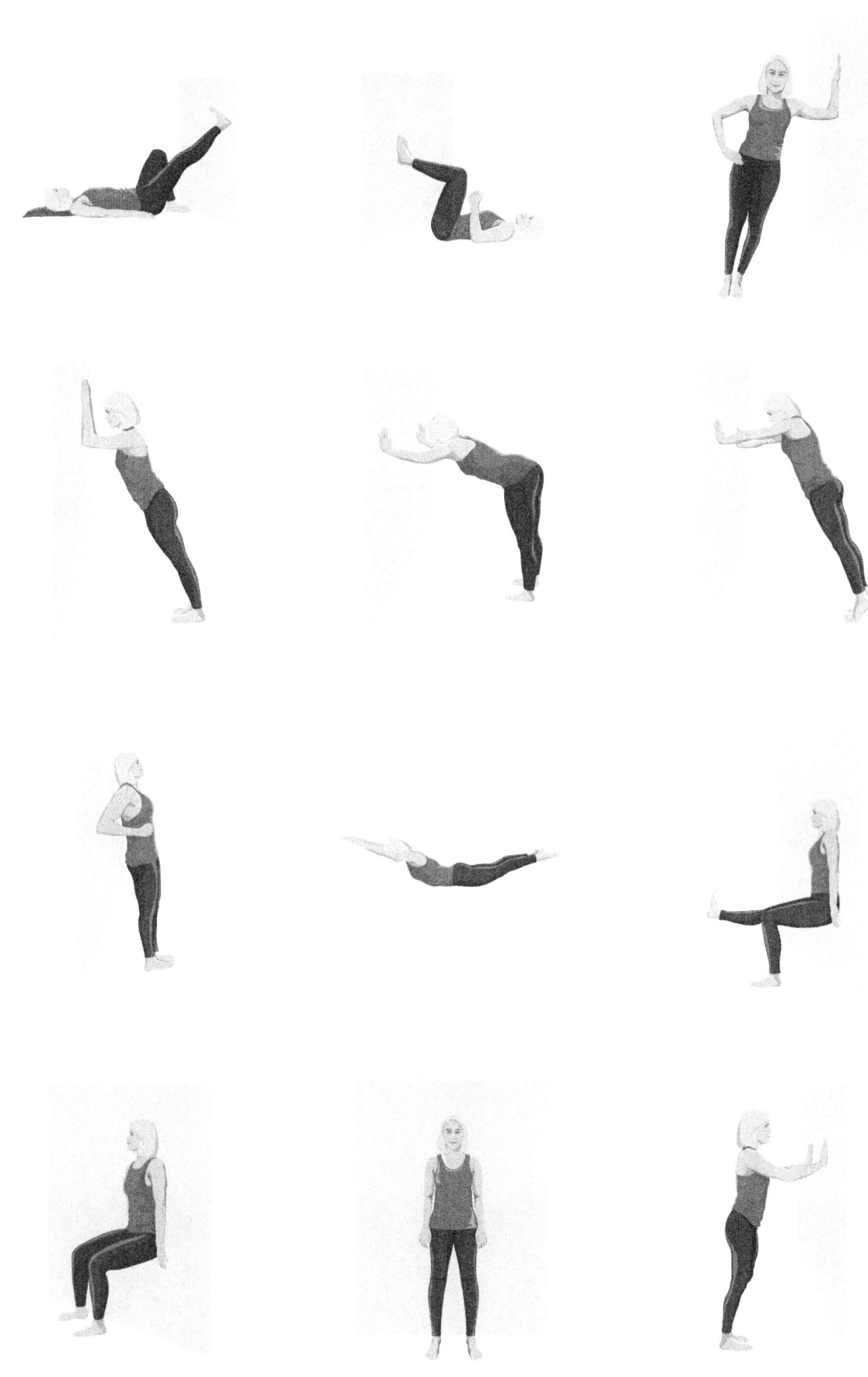

WALL PILATES WORKOUTS

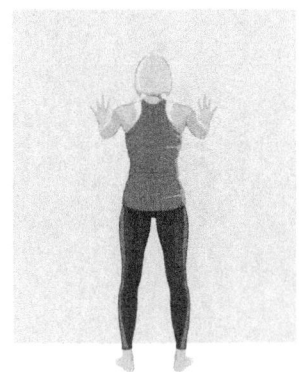 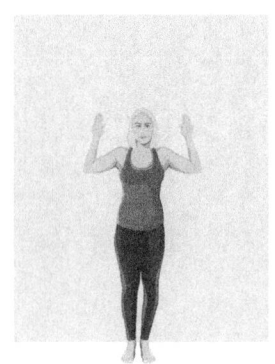 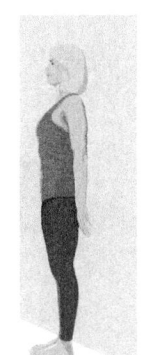
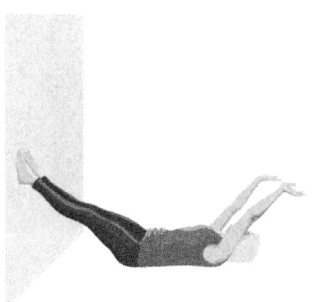

INTRODUCTION

Dear reader,

Welcome to the world of Wall Pilates! I am delighted to share my passion for this transformative exercise system with you. My name is Lisa Madison, and I have dedicated the past fifteen years of my life to teaching and practicing Pilates, with a special focus on the incredible benefits of Wall Pilates.

I have always been drawn to the power of movement and its ability to enhance our overall well-being. As a personal trainer, witnessing the positive changes in people's lives has been my greatest joy. From the very beginning of my journey, I fell in love with Pilates and its remarkable impact on the mind, body, and spirit. But it was when I discovered Wall Pilates that I truly felt the potential to take my clients' transformations to new heights.

Flexibility, tonification, and posture are areas that can greatly impact our daily lives. Throughout my years of teaching Pilates and Wall Pilates, I have witnessed countless individuals experience remarkable improvements in these aspects. The flexibility gained through Wall Pilates allows for graceful movement and ease in everyday activities. The tonification achieved empowers individuals to feel strong, confident, and ready to take on any challenge. And the postural enhancements bring a newfound sense of alignment and balance to their lives.

One of the greatest rewards for me as a teacher is witnessing the joy and empowerment that my clients experience. Whether they are beginners just starting their fitness journey or seasoned practitioners seeking to deepen their practice, Wall Pilates has been a catalyst for their transformation. I have witnessed individuals regain their confidence, overcome physical limitations, and discover newfound strength they never thought possible.

In this book, I have carefully crafted a 28-day challenge guide that will take you on a transformative journey. It is designed to help you improve flexibility, enhance tonification, and achieve optimal posture. With step-by-step exercises, an exercise chart, and expert tips, you will have all the tools necessary to embark on this empowering adventure.

Remember, this journey is not just about physical changes but also about embracing a mindset of self-care, self-discovery, and self-love. Wall Pilates has the potential to touch every aspect of your life, allowing you to uncover your inner strength and embrace the joy of movement.

Join me as we delve into the world of Wall Pilates and unlock the amazing potential that lies within you. Let us begin this transformative journey together!

With warmth and excitement,
Lisa Madison

WALL PILATES BENEFITS

Before we begin our 28-day challenge, let's look together at why adding even a few minutes a day of Wall Pilates to your routine will help you improve your relationship with your body and thus your life.

1. Accessibility

There isn't much chance that a Pilates machine will fit in a typical living room. But a barrier? That's something else. All you need to do wall Pilates is enough room to lay down with your arms outstretched. This means that almost anyone can do it.

It's a very cheap way to get all of Pilates' benefits without spending a lot of money.

Last but not least, you can still do Pilates when you're on vacation or travelling for business. All you need is a wall.

2. More Core Strenght

The core is called the "powerhouse" of the body for a reason. It helps keep the spine and pelvis stable, and it's an important part of almost every action we make.

The core is made up of the abs, obliques, hip, and lower back muscles. When you do Pilates movements, all of these muscles are used. By using your own weight and the force of the wall, you can work out all of the core muscles, not just the ab.

3. Better Spinal Alignment

One of the main goals of Pilates is to get your spine to be in the right place. This means that the spine's normal curves are in place and that the pelvis is level. When the spine is in the right place, it can support the body's weight and move more easily. On the other hand, poor balance can cause pain and stiffness.

Wall Pilates is a great way to get your back in better shape. The exercises help the spine get longer and more flexible, which can help lessen any curvature that is already there.

4. Pain Relief for the Back

Text neck, bowed shoulders, and pain in the lower back are all too common these days, and bad posture is to blame. Pilates, however, can help with all of these problems.

Pilates movements that use the wall help lengthen the spine and take pressure off the vertebrae. They also strengthen the muscles that support the spine, which can help avoid pain in the future. If your back hurts, wall Pilates is a great way to feel better.

5. Less chance of getting hurt

One of the main reasons people get hurt is because of muscle issues. When some muscles are much weaker than others, they can put too much pressure on the tendons and joints.

Pilates routines help even out muscle groups that aren't working together as well as they should. Because of this, you'll be less likely to get hurt.

Wall Pilates is especially good for people who get hurt easily. The wall gives you support and steadiness, which can help you avoid putting stress on muscles that are already weak or hurt.

6. Energy Boost

Pilates is based on how you work with your breath. In fact, a lot of the exercises are meant to teach you how to breathe better and deeper.

This deep breathing helps the blood get more oxygen and helps the blood flow better. It also calms the nervous system, which can give you more energy.

7. Better sense of body position

The body's ability to know where it is in space is called proprioception. It's what lets you touch your nose with your eyes closed or walk without looking at your feet. Athletes need to be very aware of where their bodies are in space because it can help them avoid getting hurt.

Wall Pilates routines help improve proprioception because they make you stay in control and keep your balance. You'll get a better idea of where your body is in space as you move it in different directions. This can help you escape getting hurt on the field and off.

8. Stress Relief

It's more important than ever to find ways to relax in today's fast-paced world. Exercise is a great way to do this because it helps the body make endorphins, which are chemicals that make you feel good.

Wall Pilates is a great way to relieve stress because it is soft and has low impact. The tasks make you think about yourself, which can help clear your mind and make you feel better.

9. Relief From Menstrual Pain

For women, Wall Pilates can help if you have cramps during your period. The movements can help relieve pain by stretching the muscles in the pelvis and lower back. They also increase blood flow to the area, which can help lessen swelling.

10. More Freedom of movement and flexibility

People often forget the difference between flexibility and movement and use the two words interchangeably. Think of a rubber band. It can stretch and bend. It doesn't break when stretched or pulled in different ways. Now think of a steel rod, which doesn't bend. It's not flexible and doesn't move around much.

For example, a person with good shoulder movement can lift their arms above their head and touch their shoulder blades together. If your shoulders don't move well, you might not be able to raise your arms past 90 degrees.

Flexibility and mobility can both be improved with wall Pilates routines. The stretches help the muscles get longer and give the joints a wider range of motion. This can make it easier and more free for you to move around.

11. Better flow of blood

Poor blood flow can cause tiredness, swelling, and varicose veins, among other things. Wall Pilates movements can help improve circulation by making you breathe deeply and getting fluids moving through your body.

The movements can also help strengthen the muscles around the veins, which can improve blood flow and lower the risk of getting varicose veins.

12. Better Circulation

The gentle movements that are needed for wall Pilates can help massage the organs and get the digestive system going. This can help with constipation, gas, and bloating.

The better blood flow can also help bring more oxygen and nutrients to the cells, which can help them heal and give you more energy.

13. Boosted Immune System

The immune system can be helped by exercise, and wall Pilates is no different. The workouts require you to take deep breaths, which helps your lungs work better and lets you take in more oxygen. This can help you stay healthy and fight off infections.

14. Bones with more mass

Osteoporosis is a disease that makes bones less dense and makes them more likely to break. It happens most often in older adults, but people of all ages can get it. One of the best ways to avoid and treat osteoporosis is to exercise. This is because exercise helps build and keep bone mass.

15. Better mental performance

Cognitive loss is a normal part of getting older, but it can be sped up by things like not being active enough. Exercise has been shown to improve brain function and slow down the decrease of brain function.

Several measures of how well your brain works have gotten better, according to studies. Pilates training has been shown to lead to new neurons, more neurotransmitters, longer-lasting neurons that are important for memory and learning, and more blood flow to the brain.

16. Motivation Boost

People who want to live a busy life sometimes have trouble getting started. When you don't see results right away or when your workout routine gets boring, it can be hard to stay inspired.

Wall Pilates can help boost drive by giving you a new and difficult way to work out. You can also change the movements to make them easier or harder, depending on what you need. This lets you eventually make your workouts harder as you get stronger and healthier.

Having a strong pelvic floor has been linked to a better quality of life and more sexual pleasure in multiple studies. The pelvic floor muscles help support the bladder and other parts inside the body, and they tighten when a person is sexually active.

Pilates can help players do better by making them stronger, more flexible, and giving them a wider range of motion. Balance and coordination can also be helped by the activities.

Golf, tennis, basketball, and football are some of the most famous sports that can be helped by wall Pilates. Golfers can get stronger and have a wider range of motion, and tennis players can improve their balance and agility.

Pilates can help you sleep better at night if you do it once a week. Deep breathing exercises and relaxation methods can help calm the mind and body. They can also help reduce stress. This can lead to better and more restful sleep.

Wall Pilates can help pregnant women in many of the same ways that it helps other people. Strength, flexibility, and range of motion can all be improved by doing the routines. They can also help improve rhythm and balance.

Pilates can also help get the body ready for labor and birth. Deep breathing exercises can help calm the mind and body, and pelvic floor movements can help strengthen the muscles used during childbirth.

Pilates is a great workout for pregnant women because it can be changed to fit different stages of pregnancy. The intensity can be turned up or down as needed, and the workouts can be changed so that the body doesn't have to work too hard.

28-DAYS CALLENGE

It's time to roll up our sleeves and start having fun. I fully understand how busy you may feel from your daily commitments; all I ask is for you to take 5–10 minutes a day for the next 28 days. At the end of the challenge, feel free to go back to the benefits section to verify that it wasn't humbug!

Each day I will explain a new exercise; it will be up to you to choose whether to limit yourself to its execution or to add even 1-2 exercises among those explained before the last one.

Let's get started!

DAYS 1-5
Are you ready? Let's go!
WALL CALF STRETCH

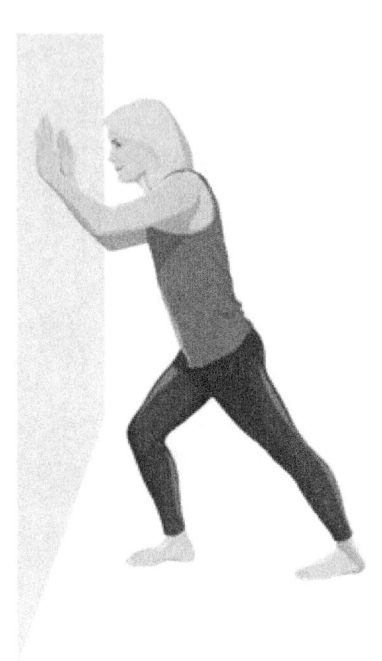

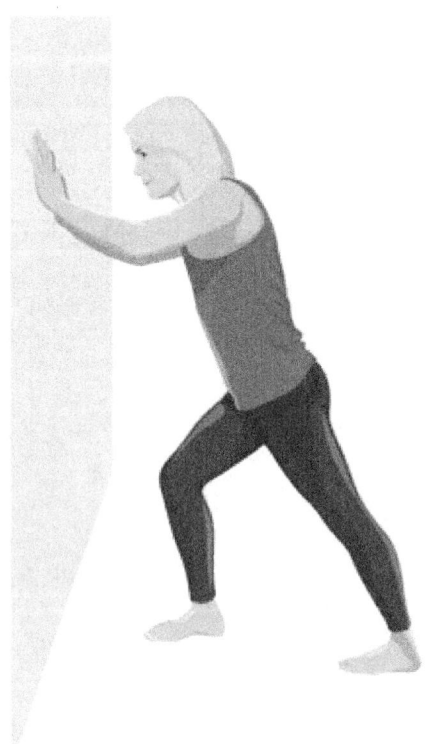

The wall calf stretch helps increase ankle mobility, strengthens calves, and reduces the risk of ankle injuries.

INSTRUCTIONS:

1. Place both hands on a wall and face the wall for stability. Start with one foot away from the wall and go forward until both feet are several inches behind the wall.
2. You should be able to feel a stretch in the calf muscle of your rear leg as you press your body forward while keeping both heels planted on the ground in step 2.
3. Three, maintain this position for 15-30 seconds before releasing and alternating sides.
4. Perform numerous sets on each side, paying special attention to maintaining deep, steady breathing.

- Maintain a strong abdominal contraction and a straight spine during the entire exercise.
- Keep your knee in front of your toes.
- Step your front foot farther away from the wall to increase the intensity of the stretch.

WALL CHEST STRETCH

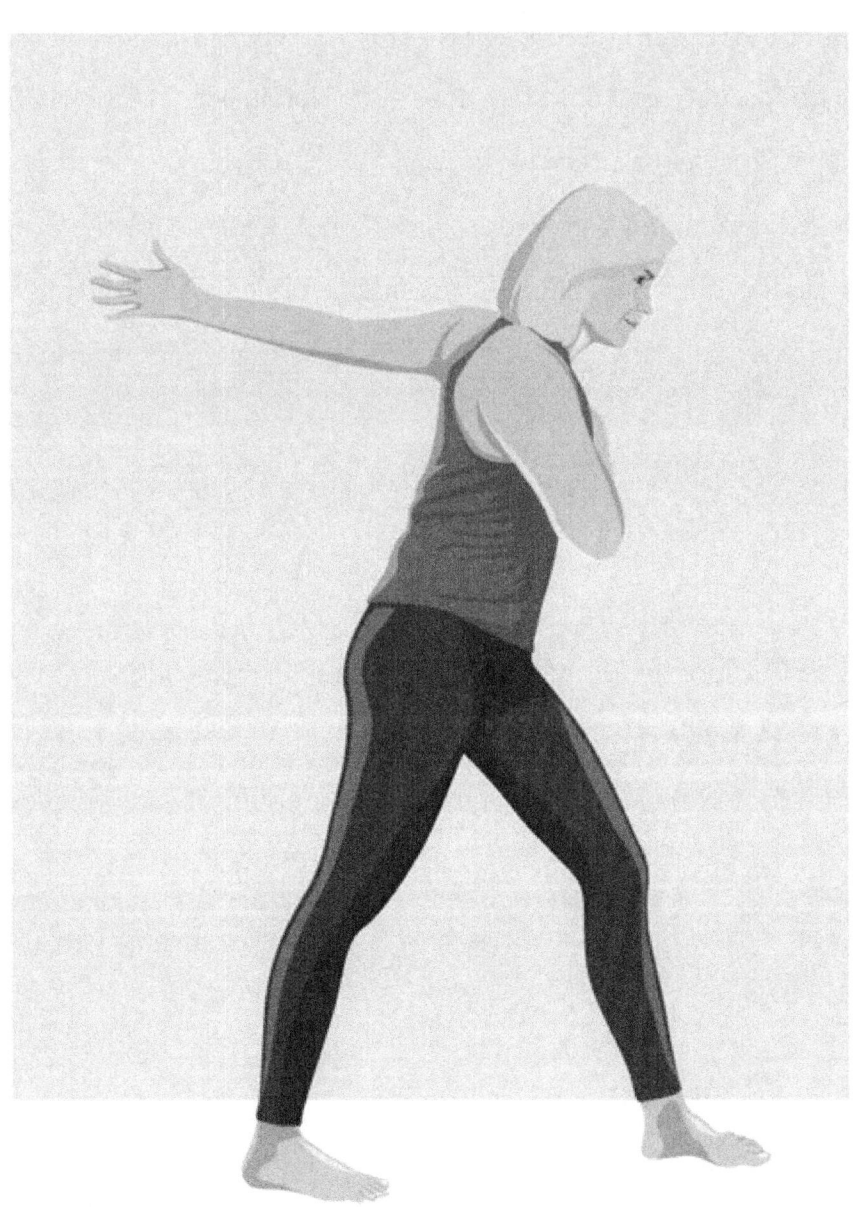

The Wall Chest Stretch is a great way to stretch the shoulders, arms, and upper back and open up the chest. It is perfect for people who sit or hunch over a desk for long periods of time.

INSTRUCTIONS:

1. Stand facing the wall and put your hands on it with your elbows bent at shoulder height.
2. Take a step back and lean into the wall, keeping your feet hip-width apart.
3. Let your chest fall toward the wall, and feel your chest and shoulders stretch.
4. Hold the stretch for 20 to 30 seconds while breathing deeply.
5. Move away from the wall slowly and let go of the stretch.

- During the stretch, keep your shoulders loose and down.
- When you lean forward, don't let your lower back rise.
- Breathe in and out slowly and deeply to help you relax into the stretch.
- Change: To make the stretch stronger, put your hands higher on the wall. You can also stretch your wrists by turning your palms up.
- Don't overstretch and pay attention to what your body can handle.

WALL SQUAT

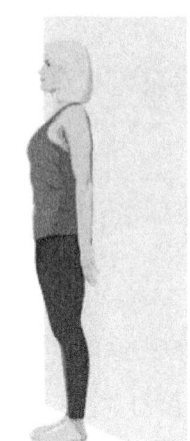

1.

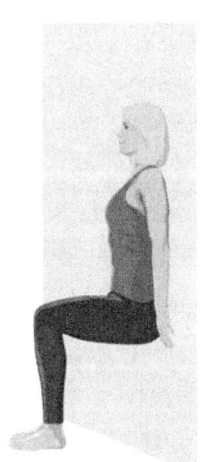

2.

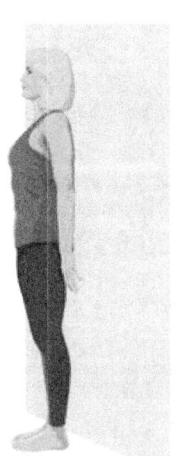

3.

The wall squat is a resistance workout that strengthens and tones the muscles in the legs, glutes, and core. It also makes your stance and balance better.

INSTRUCTIONS:

1. Stand with your back to the wall and your feet about hip-width apart. Use your core muscles and don't tense up your shoulders.
2. Slide your back down the wall slowly until your legs are parallel to the floor. Make sure your knees are exactly over your ankles and that your weight is evenly spread between your feet.
3. Stay here for a few deep breaths. Keep your back flat against the wall and your core muscles engaged.
4. Push slowly through your feet to get back up. Make sure to keep your form the same throughout the whole move.

- If it's hard for you to stay in the squat position for a few breaths, start by keeping it for a few seconds. As you get stronger, keep adding time to it.
- Hold a weight in each hand or wrap a resistance band around your thighs to make the workout harder.
- Keep your knees in line with your toes to keep your knees from getting too tired.

WALL LUNGE

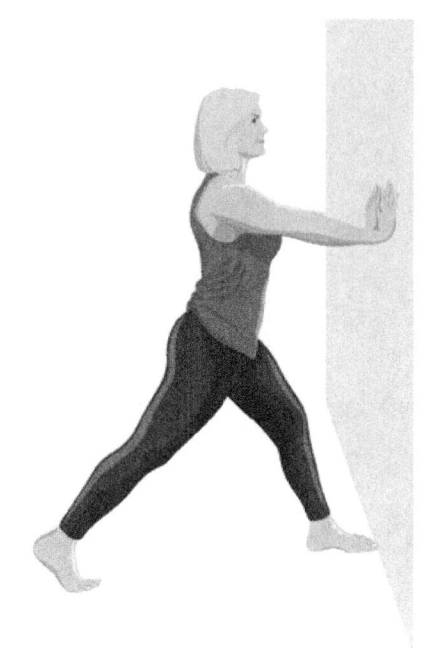

1.

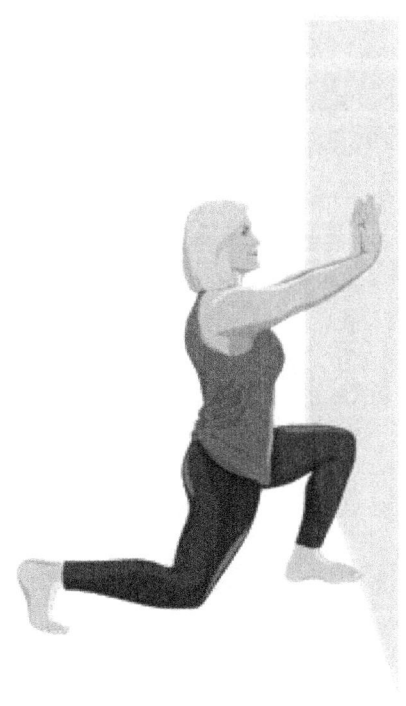

2.

The quads, hamstrings, and glutes may all be worked on while increasing your balance and coordination with wall lunges.

INSTRUCTIONS:

1. Place your feet hip-width apart as you stand facing the wall.
2. Place your hands at shoulder height on the wall.
3. Take one step back and rest your toe against the wall.
4. While keeping your front knee directly over your ankle, lower your rear knee toward the ground.
5. Push yourself back up to where you started, utilizing the wall for stability and support.
6. After a few repetitions, switch legs and resume the exercise.

- To maintain good form and balance throughout the exercise, keep your core engaged.
- To prevent knee discomfort, make sure your front knee is directly above your ankle.
- Start with a shorter step back if you have balance issues, or lean on a chair for support.

WALL SIDE LEG EXTENSION

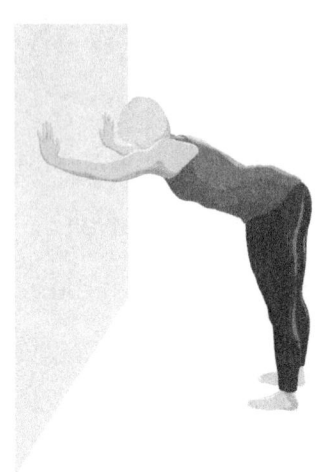

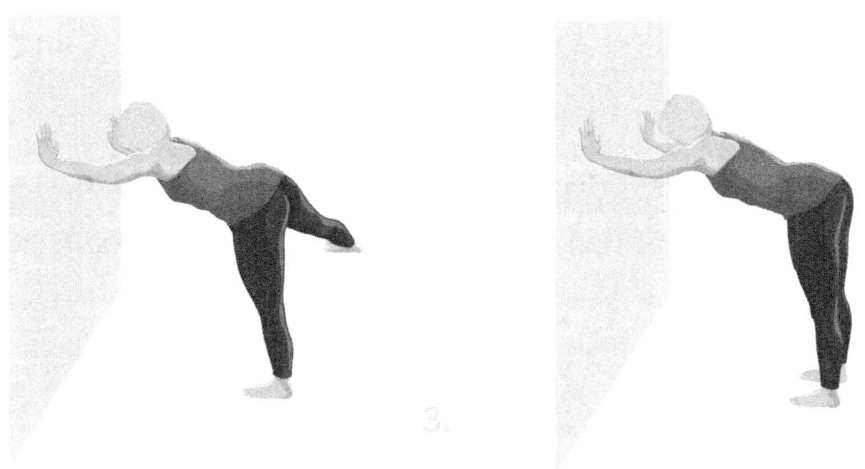

The glutes, hips, and outside thighs are the areas worked by the wall side leg extension exercise. It is excellent for enhancing the stability and lower body strength.

INSTRUCTIONS:

1. Place your left hand on the wall while standing with your left side facing the wall.
2. Keeping your right foot firmly planted on the ground, take a tiny left foot step away from the wall.
3. With your right leg raised straight out to the side and your toes pointed front, contract your core muscles.
4. After maintaining the position for a few while, carefully drop your leg back to the ground.
5. Continue as many times as necessary (e.g. 12), then switch sides.

- To ensure stability, keep your standing leg slightly bent.

Throughout the exercise, maintain a forward-facing hip position.

- To increase stability, contract your core muscles and squeeze your glutes.

Place your hand on the lower portion of the wall or wrap a resistance band around your ankles to make the workout simpler. Use ankle weights or up the amount of repetitions to make it more difficult.

DAYS 6-10

Congratulations on completing the first five days of the Wall Pilates Challenge! Your consistency and dedication to this practice are admirable, and you should be proud of yourself for making it this far.

As you continue with the challenge, there may be times when you feel like giving up or skipping a day. However, I encourage you to keep going and stay committed to the program. Remember that the benefits of Wall Pilates come with consistency and patience, and the results will be worth it.

WALL KNEE FOLDS

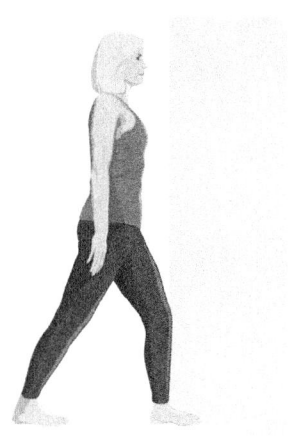

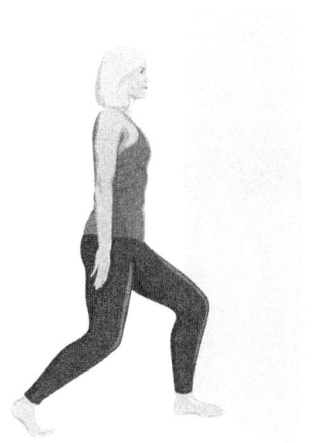
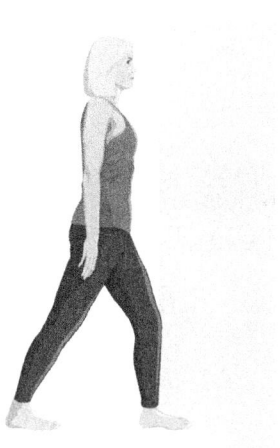

Lower abs and hip flexors are worked during the difficult exercise known as wall knee folds.

INSTRUCTIONS:

1. Lie on your back with your feet flat against the wall and your hips about a foot away.
2. Lay your hands at your sides with the palms facing the ground.
3. Contract your abdominal muscles and raise your head and shoulders off the floor.
4. With your knees bent and your feet flat against the wall, slowly glide your feet down the wall toward your hips.
5. Remain in the position for a moment, then slowly return to your starting position by sliding your feet up the wall.
6. Carry out 10 to 15 repetitions.

- To preserve your lower back, keep your core engaged throughout the workout.
- Maintain a flat back against the wall at all times.
- Keep your form by moving slowly and deliberately.

WALL SCISSOR KICKS

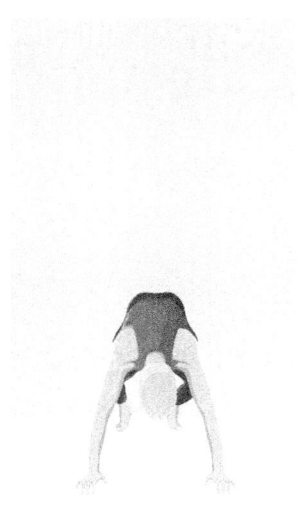

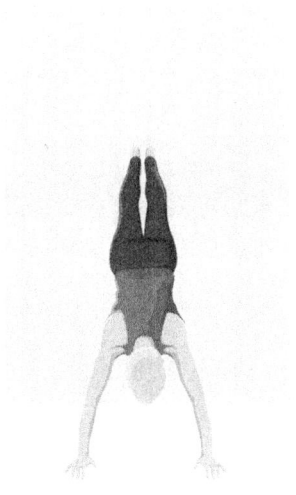

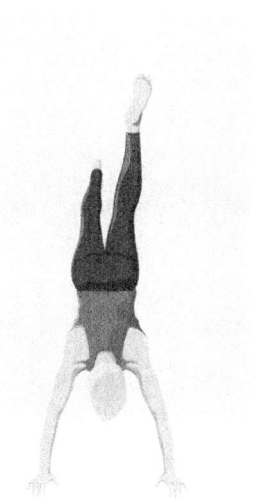

Exercises that challenge the lower abdomen, hip flexors, and inner thighs include wall scissor kicks.

INSTRUCTIONS:

1. Lie on your back with your legs extended straight up against the wall and your hips about a foot away from the wall.
2. Lay your hands at your sides with the palms facing the ground.
3. Contract your abdominal muscles and raise your head and shoulders off the floor.
4. While keeping your right leg straight up against the wall, stoop your left leg down toward the floor.
5. Point your toes in the direction of your head as you lower your leg.
6. Lift your left foot back up to the beginning position just before touching the ground. Repeat on the other side.
7. Perform ten to fifteen repetitions on each leg.

- To protect your lower back, keep your core engaged throughout the workout.
- Keep your toes pointing in the direction of your head and keep your legs as straight as you can.
- Keep your form by moving slowly and deliberately.

WALL PUSH-UPS

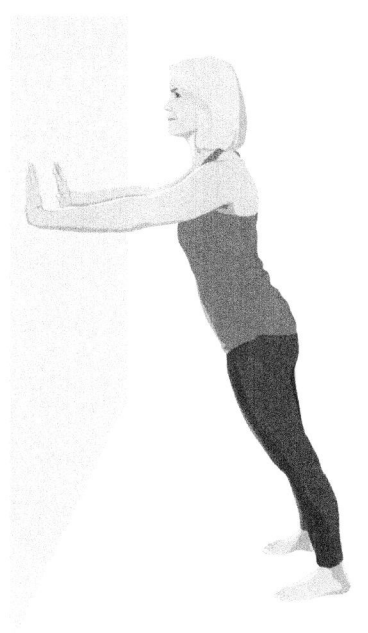

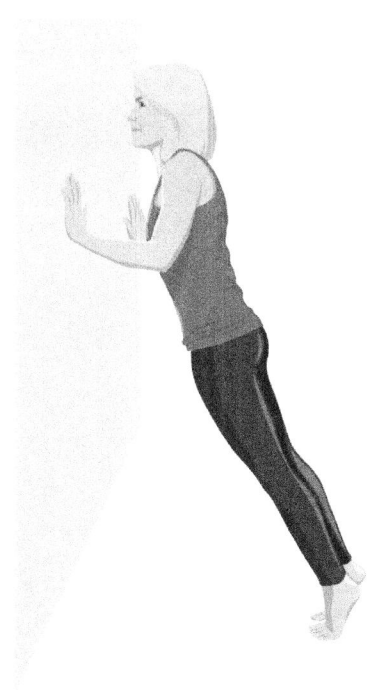

Push-ups against a wall work the triceps, shoulders, and chest muscles. Strength and endurance in the upper body are increased.

INSTRUCTIONS:

1. Place your hands flat against the wall at shoulder height while standing facing the wall with your arms out in front of you.
2. Take a step back until your arms are straight and your body is at a little angle.
3. Lower your chest toward the wall while bending your elbows.
4. Return to the beginning posture by pushing back up while maintaining core stability.
5. Repeat for a predetermined period of time, or for 10 to 15 repetitions.

- Keep your elbows close to your body and your hands shoulder-width apart.
- To keep your back from arching, keep your core muscles tight.
- Pay close attention to maintaining your balance against the wall at all times.

WALL ARM CIRCLES

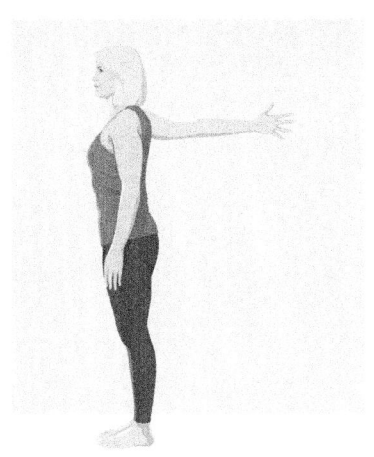
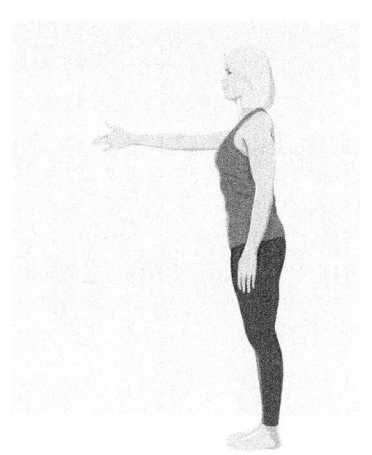
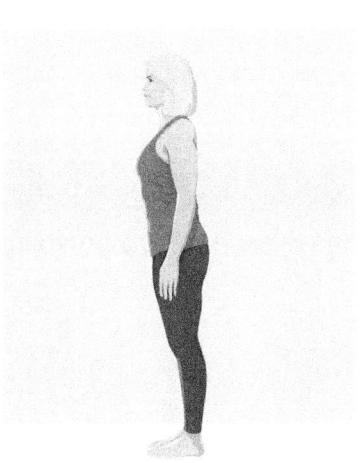
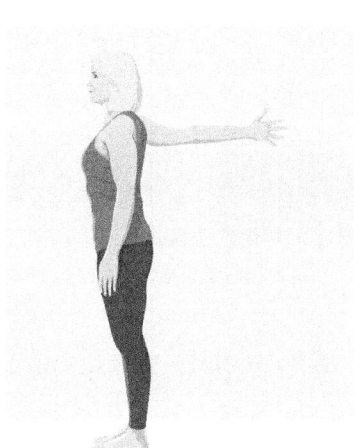

Wall arm circles targets the shoulders and arms in particular to strengthen and tone the upper body. Additionally, this exercise can increase upper back and shoulder flexibility.

INSTRUCTIONS:

1. Stand with your back to the wall, feet hip-width apart, and arms out in front of you at shoulder height.
2. With your fingers pointing up, place your hands on the wall shoulder-width apart and at shoulder height.
3. While maintaining a straight arm position, move your arms slowly in small circles by moving them 10-15 times ahead and then 10-15 times backward.
4. Attempt to maintain a relaxed posture and refrain from hunching your shoulders up toward your ears.
5. Pay attention to maintaining smooth, controlled movement.

- Begin with smaller circles and progressively enlarge them as you gain self-assurance and comfort.
- you maintain stability and control during the exercise, make sure you use your core muscles.
- Adjust the size and speed of your circles if you feel any pain or discomfort, or speak with a healthcare provider.

WALL HIGH KICKS

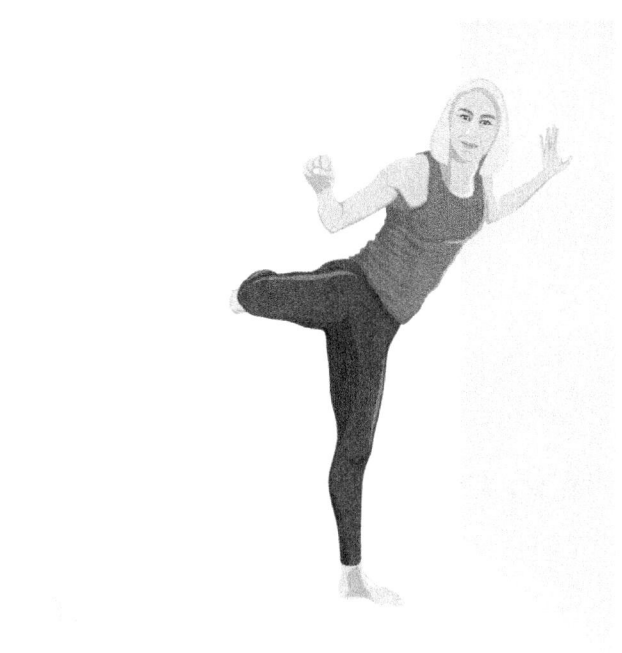

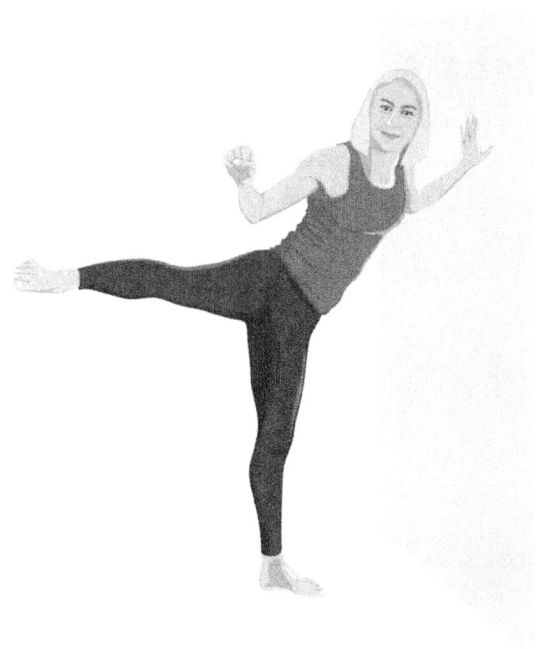

This workout focuses on the lower body, especially the glutes, hip flexors, and quads. Additionally, it enhances balance and flexibility.

INSTRUCTIONS:

1. Place your palms at shoulder height against the wall while standing facing the wall with your feet hip-distance apart.
2. With your right leg raised, straight and toes flexed, engage your core muscles.
3. As high as you can lift your leg without endangering your balance or body alignment, kick it up toward the ceiling.
4. Reposition your leg to the starting position slowly.
5. Do the same thing with your left leg.
6. Switch legs and perform a total of 10 to 15 repetitions.

- To maintain stability, keep your standing leg straight and firmly planted on the ground.
- When kicking your leg up, try not to arch your back or lean forward.

DAYS 11-15

Here you can find exercises for Days 11-15 of the 28-day Wall Pilates Challenge. You should be proud of how far you've come. Here we'll continue our journey of wall-based exercises, with the goal of improving your strength, flexibility, and balance. The daily schedule is designed to help you advance at your own speed by building on the groundwork you've already laid. So, let's get started on your exciting new Wall Pilates workouts and continue your path to better health and vitality!

WALL OBLIQUE TWISTS

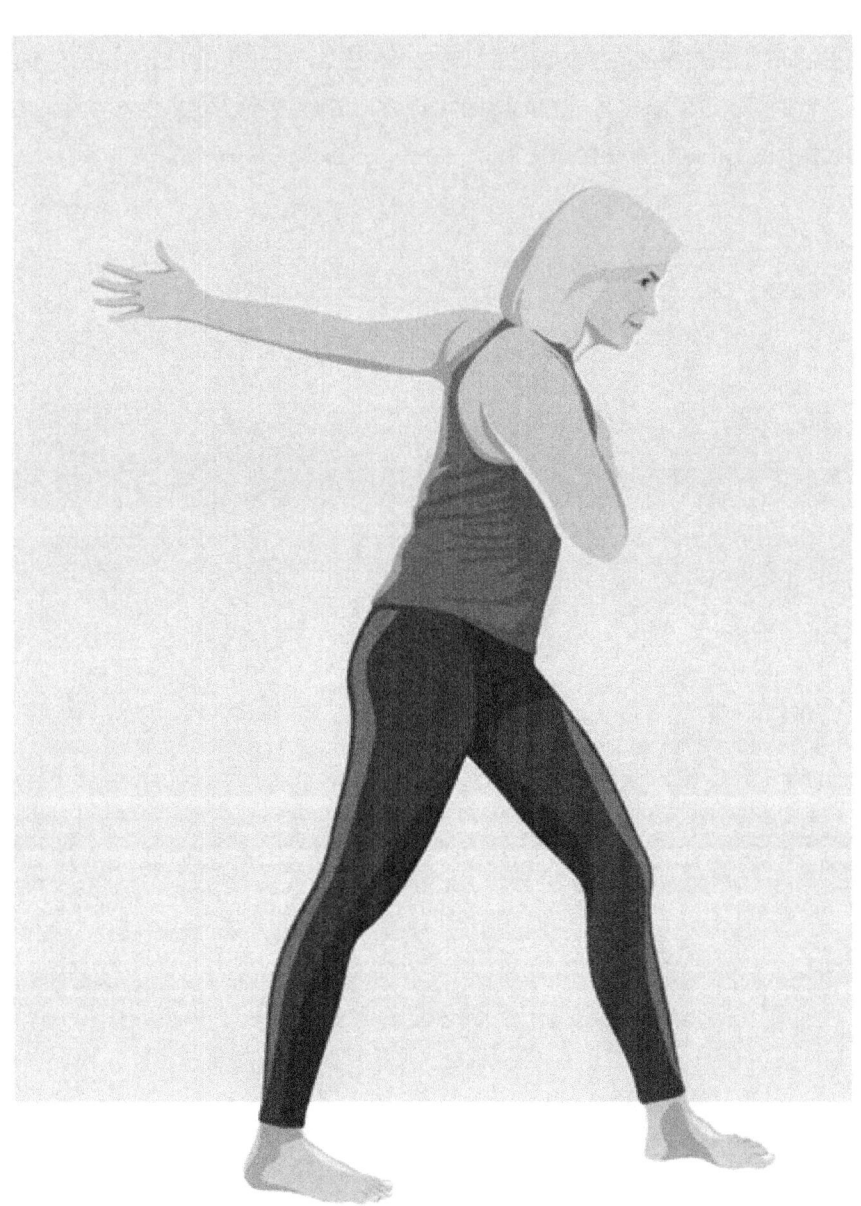

The oblique muscles, which are on the sides of the abdomen, are the focus of this exercise. It enhances spinal mobility and tones and strengthens the core.

INSTRUCTIONS:

1. Place your hands on the wall at shoulder height while standing with your side towards the wall.
2. Take a step away from the wall with your feet and raise your arms straight in front of you.
3. Turn your torso to the left while contracting your abdominal muscles, pushing your right elbow up near your left knee.
4. At the bottom of the movement, take a little pause before returning to the starting position.
5. On the other side, repeat.
6. For a total of 10-15 repetitions, switch sides.

- Throughout the workout, maintain an elevated chest and an extended spine.
- Instead than only using your arms to rotate, concentrate on doing so from your ribcage.

WALL PIKE

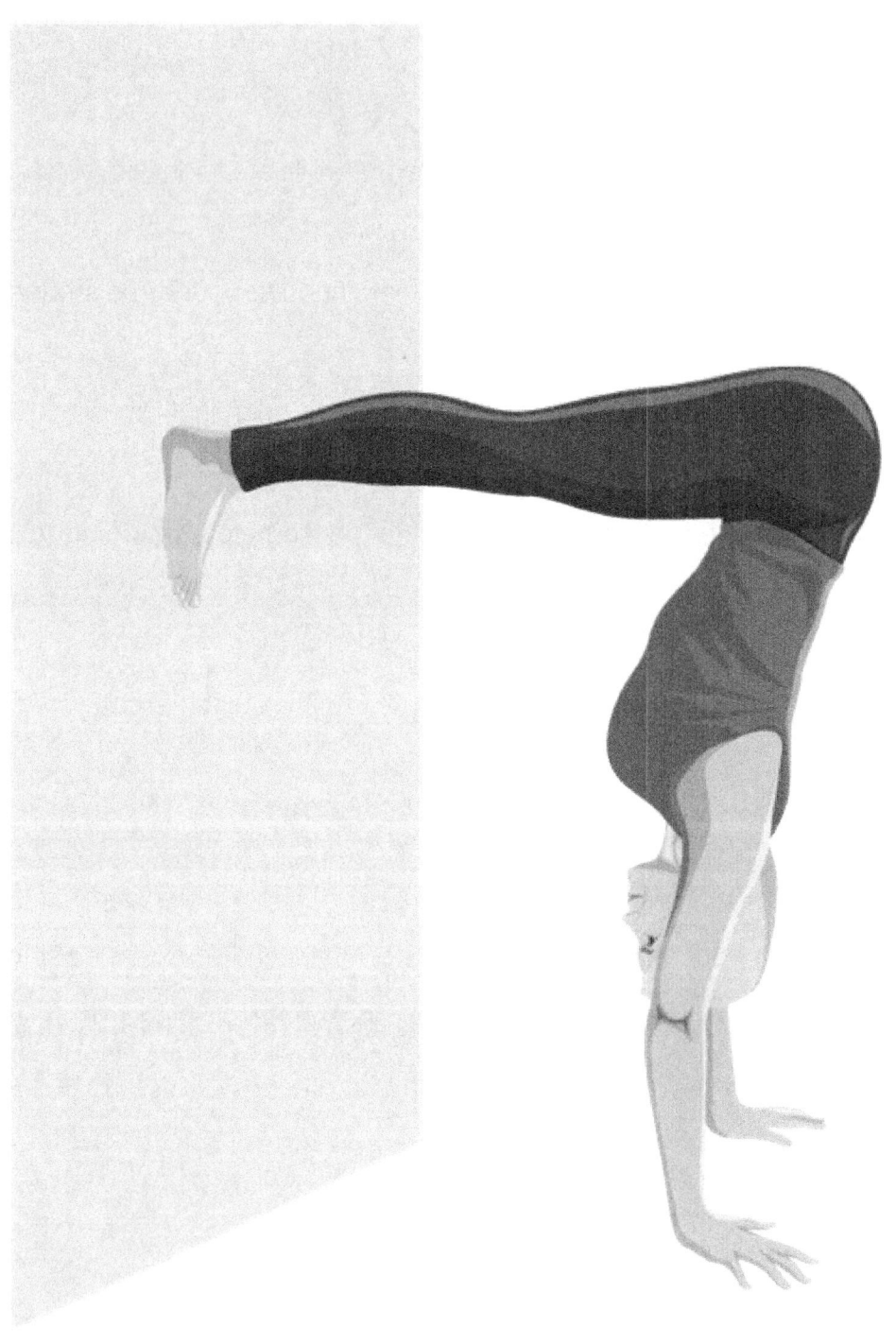

The core, shoulders, and hip flexors are the focus of the Wall Pike workout. It is excellent for enhancing flexibility, shoulder stability, and core strength.

INSTRUCTIONS:

1. Place your feet against the wall and your hands on the floor in a push-up posture to begin.
2. Climb the wall with your feet until your hips are raised and your body is shaped like an inverted V.
3. While maintaining your arms and legs straight, contract your core muscles and lift your hips as high as you can toward the ceiling.

- As you perform the exercise, maintain straight arms and legs.
- Keep your shoulders down and relaxed.
- Pay attention to engaging your abs to raise your hips upward.
- Reduce the angle of the pike by walking your feet higher up the wall to make the workout simpler. Increase the difficulty by moving your feet closer to the wall or by adding a push-up at the base of the pike.

WALL HAMSTRING STRETCH

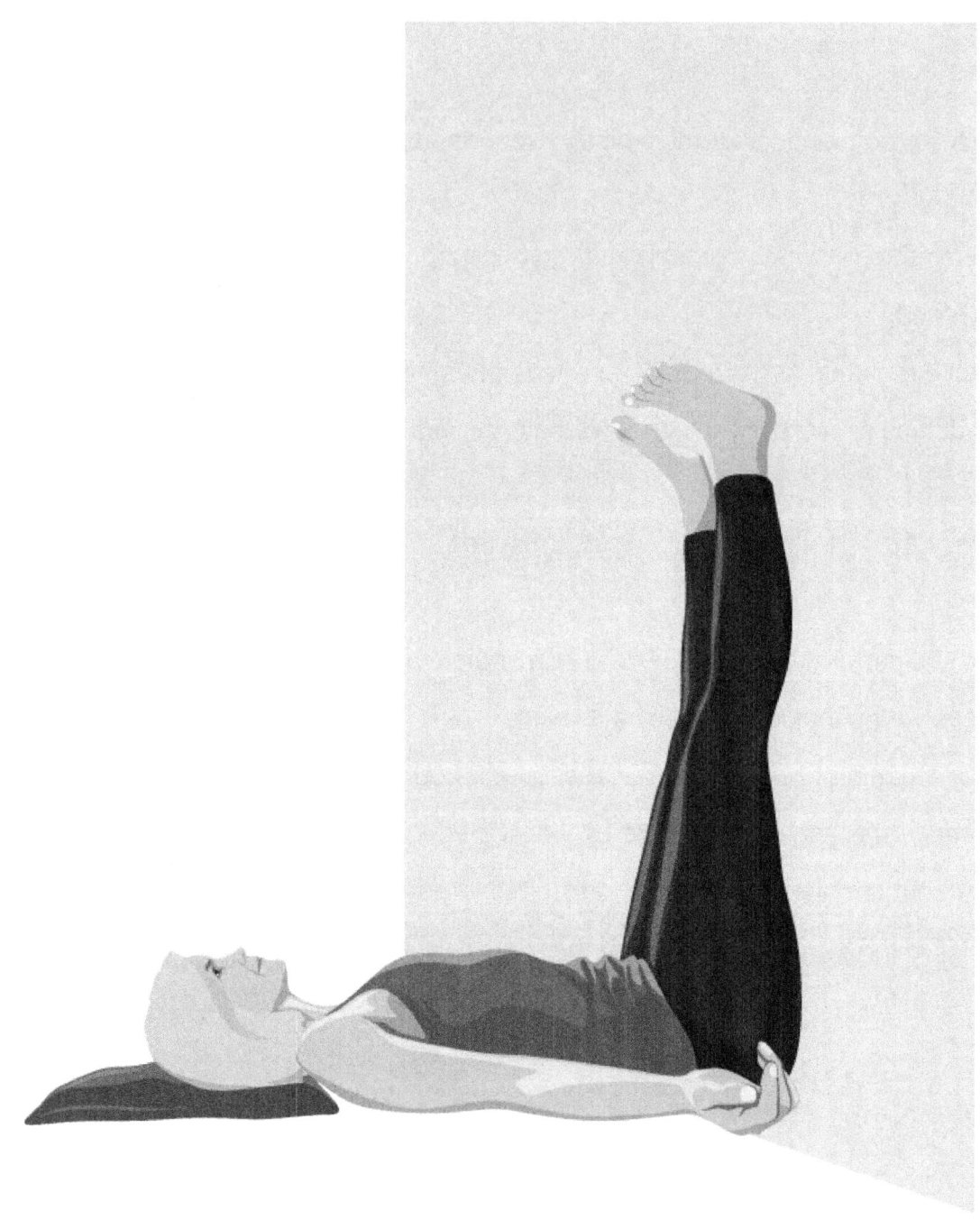

Your hamstrings and lower back can become more flexible with the wall hamstring stretch. For people who spend a lot of time sitting and want to combat the detrimental consequences of a sedentary lifestyle, this stretch is ideal.

INSTRUCTIONS:

1. Place your hips close to the wall while lying on your back with your legs straight.
2. Lift one leg slowly, keeping your knee slightly bent, and place the heel on the wall.
3. To feel a stretch in your hamstrings, gently press your heel against the wall while pushing your toes up toward your shin.
4. After holding the stretch for 30 to 60 seconds, switch legs and repeat.
5. Make careful to breathe deeply while performing the stretch, inhaling to start it and expelling to deepen it.

- If your knee is bothering you or hurting, keep it bent more or shift your hips farther away from the wall. Avoid arching your lower back and maintain a flat back against the floor.

WALL SINGLE-LEG STRETCH WALL

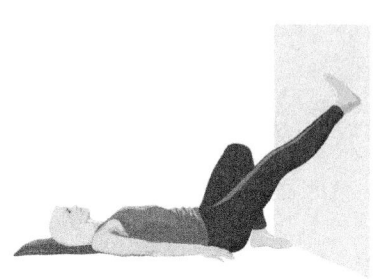

1.

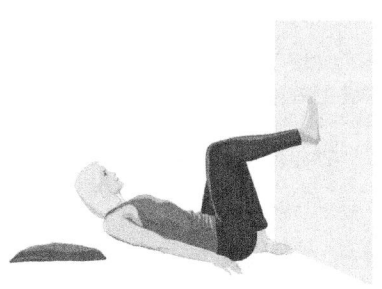

2.

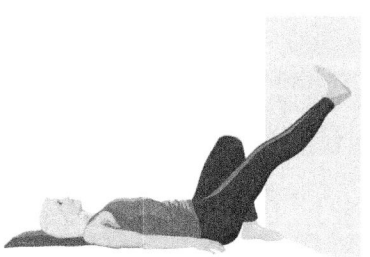

3.

The Wall Single-Leg Stretch works the abs, hips, and legs while also improving balance and core stability. By holding on to the wall, this exercise is good for people of all fitness levels and can be changed to fit different skills.

INSTRUCTIONS:

1. Start by lying on your back with your arms by your sides and your legs stretched out along the wall. Press your lower back hard into the mat and tighten your stomach muscles.
2. Keep your left leg straight along the wall and bend your right knee. Place the bottom of your right foot against the wall.
3. Inhale to get ready, and as you exhale, lift your head, neck, and shoulders off the mat and curl your upper body toward your right knee. At the same time, reach your left leg up toward the sky while keeping it against the wall.
4. Inhale to return to the starting position, bringing your head, neck, and shoulders back down to the floor and turning your right knee to put your foot back on the wall.
5. On the other side, bend your left knee and stretch your right leg up towards the sky.
6. Switch sides until you've done 8–10 reps on each leg.

- If you're a beginner or don't have much flexibility, you can start with a smaller range of motion, moving your head and shoulders off the mat without fully rolling up.

WALL HIP BRIDGE

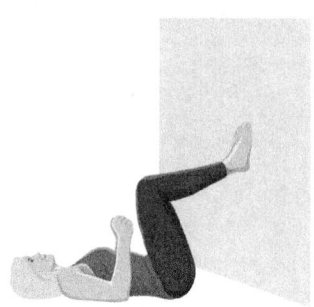

1.

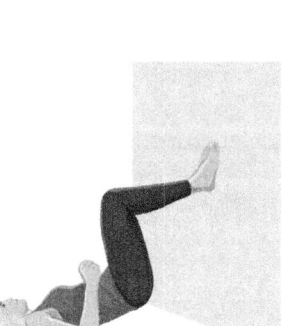

2.

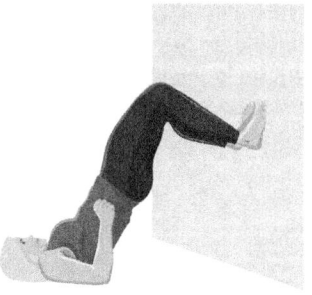

3.

Targeting your glutes, hamstrings, and lower back while enhancing your stability and posture with the wall hip bridge is a terrific exercise.

INSTRUCTIONS:

1. Face the wall while lying on your back with your feet hip-width apart and your knees bent.
2. Pushing your feet into the wall while keeping your shoulders and upper back on the floor, engage your core and lift your hips off the floor.
3. After a few period of holding the position, return your hips to the floor.
4. Focus on keeping perfect form and activating your glutes and core the entire while you repeat the movement for a few reps.

- Avoid arching your lower back during the exercise; instead, concentrate on using your glutes and core to elevate your hips.
- Keep your feet flat against the wall the entire time.

DAYS 16-20

I'm excited to see that you've reached Days 16-20 of the Wall Pilates 28-Day Challenge! You're now well into the second half of the program and should be proud of your progress in your Pilates practice. In this section, I'll be providing you with new workout options that will test your strength, flexibility, and balance, while introducing some fresh movements to keep things interesting. So, let's continue pushing ourselves and making the most of these Wall Pilates Workouts to enhance health and fitness.

WALL SIDE PLANK

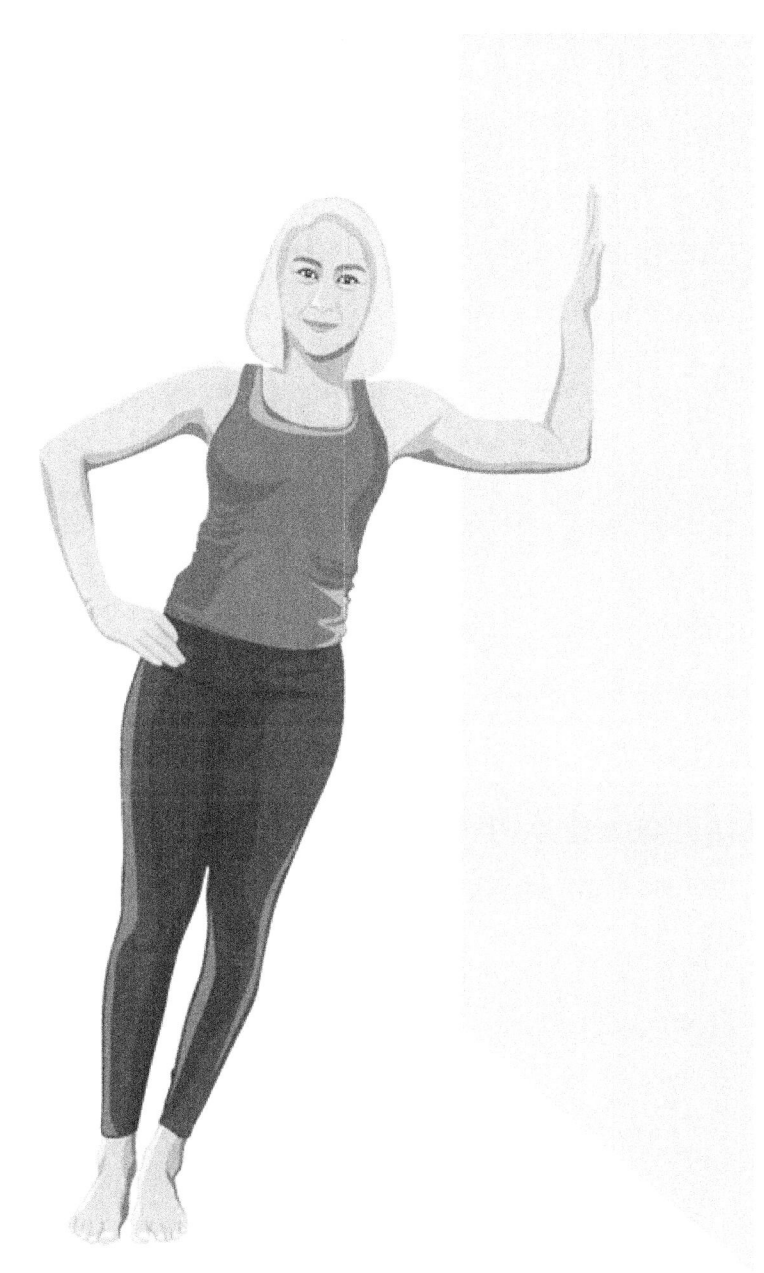

The wall side plank is a fantastic exercise for your obliques and for strengthening and stabilizing your entire core.

INSTRUCTIONS:

1. While standing with your side facing the wall, position your forearm at shoulder height on the wall.
2. Take a backward step so that your body is straight from head to heels.
3. To create a straight line from your head to your heels, engage your core and lift your hips off the floor.
4. Maintain the position for 30 to 60 seconds, then swap sides and do it again.

- To ensure appropriate form, keep your core engaged throughout the exercise.
- Throughout the workout, make sure to breathe deeply, inhaling as you get ready to lift your hips and exhaling as you do so.
- Put your top foot in front of your bottom foot for increased stability if you have difficulties staying balanced.

WALL PLANK

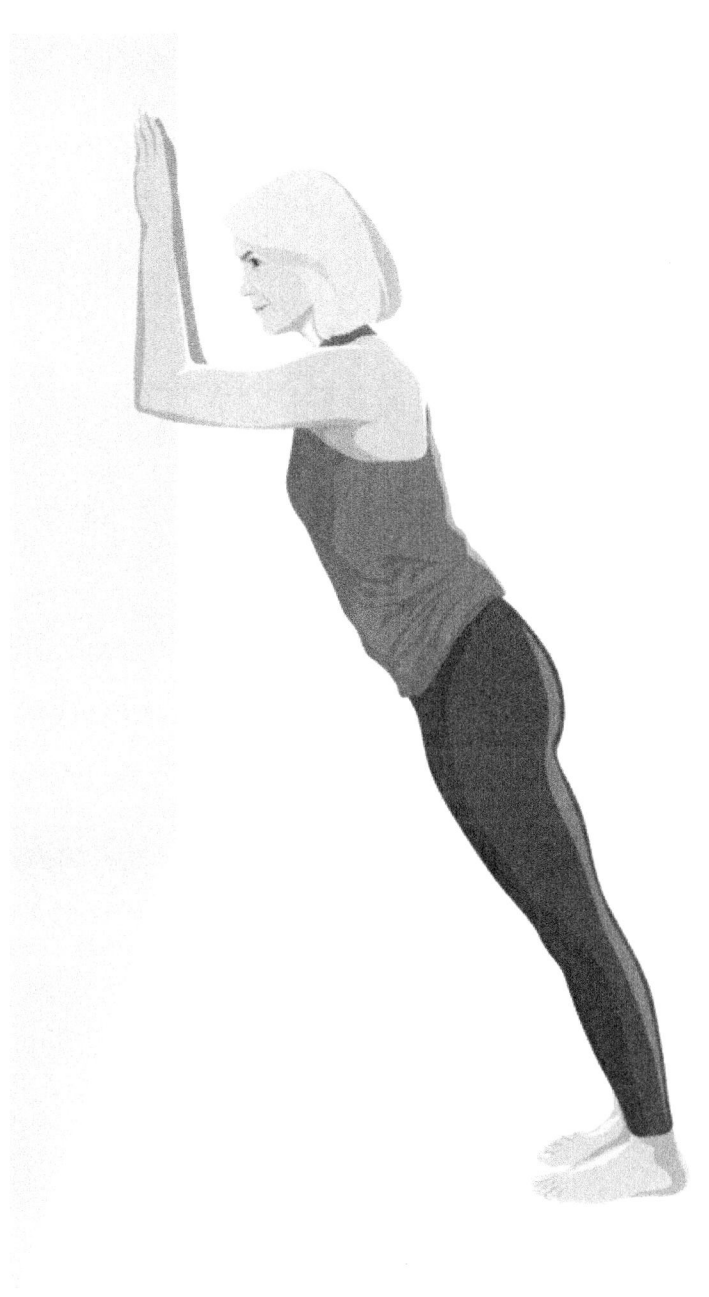

The classic plank exercise may be modified to work the abdomen, shoulders, and upper back while enhancing balance and core stability.

INSTRUCTIONS:

1. While facing the wall, raise your hands to shoulder height.
2. Retract two steps, keeping your body straight from head to heels.
3. Contract your abs and hold the posture for 30 to 60 seconds, or for as long as you are able to keep your form in tact.
4. After 30 seconds of release and rest, repeat for 2-3 sets.

- To ensure appropriate form, keep your core engaged throughout the exercise.
- Ensure that your hands are placed squarely beneath your shoulders.
- Pay attention to maintaining a straight line from your head to your heels.

WALL TRICEP DIPS

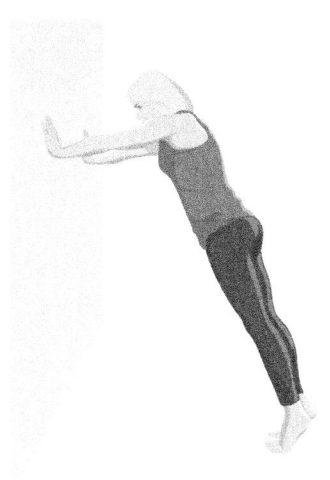

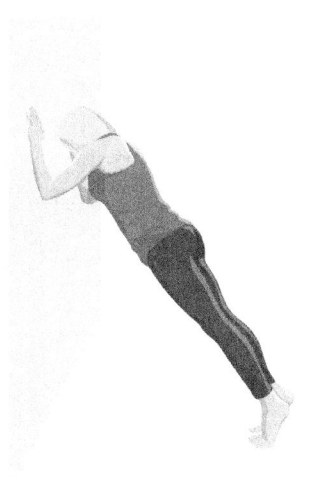
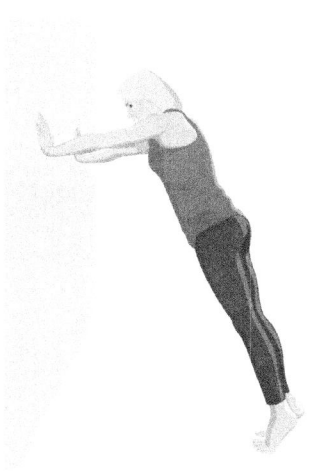

The triceps, shoulders, and core muscles are the focus of this workout. The upper body is strengthened and toned as a result.

INSTRUCTIONS:

1. With your back to the wall and your hands shoulder-width apart, stand facing away from it.
2. Advance your feet until your body is 45 degrees from the wall.
3. To lower your body toward the wall, engage your core and flex your elbows.
4. At the bottom of the movement, pause for a brief second before straightening your arms to return to the beginning position.
5. Repeat between 10 and 15 times.

- As you lower yourself, keep your elbows tight to your torso.
- Try not to hunch your shoulders up toward your ears or shrug them.

WALL REVERSE PLANK

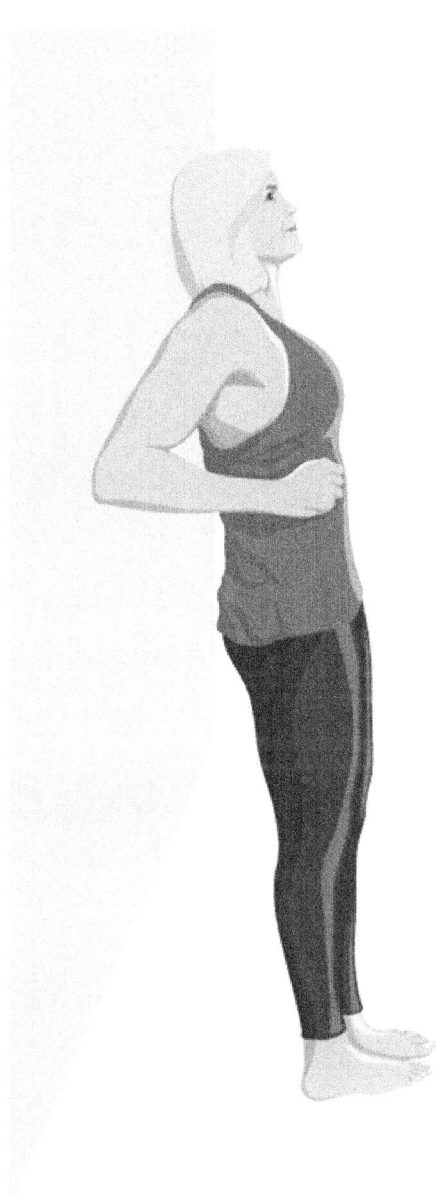

The Wall Reverse Plank works your core primarily, but it also works your glutes, hamstrings, and back.

This workout enhances your balance, stability, and posture. Your upper body and core muscles are also strengthened, which can lessen your risk of back problems and enhance your overall sports performance.

INSTRUCTIONS:

1. Start by sitting down on the floor with your legs out in front of you and your back against the wall.
2. With your fingers pointing down toward your feet, place your hands on the floor next to your hips.
3. Until your body is in a straight line from your shoulders to your heels, press through your hands and raise your hips off the ground.
4. Keep your shoulders down and away from your ears. Engage your core.
5. While maintaining the position, breathe deeply for 10 to 30 seconds.
6. To exit the pose, bring your hips back to the floor.

- To help your shoulders stay in place, keep your hands shoulder-width apart with your fingers pointing down at your feet.
- To raise your hips, contract your glutes and hamstrings; do not slouch into your lower back.
- If this pose is too challenging, you can modify by bending your knees and placing your feet flat on the ground.

WALL SUPERMAN

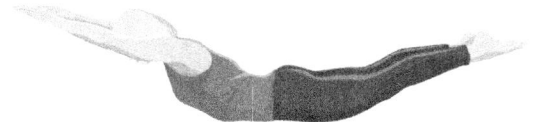

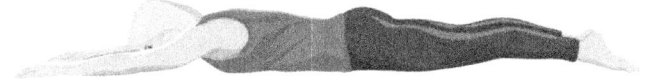

The muscles in the lower back that support the spine and enhance posture are the focus of this workout. The hamstrings and glutes are also worked.It.

INSTRUCTIONS:

1. Lay down on the floor face down with your arms out straight in front of you.
2. Squeeze the wall with your palms while contracting your abdominal muscles.
3. While maintaining your gaze fixed on the wall, raise your arms, chest, and legs as high as you can.
4. After briefly holding at the movement's peak, bring your body back to its starting position.
5. Repeat between 10 and 15 times.

- Avoid looking up or down to keep your neck in line with your spine.
- Try not to tense your shoulders or allow them to slouch forward toward your ears.

DAYS 21-25

Welcome to Days 21–25 of the 28-Day Challenge for Wall Pilates Workouts! You are a Pilates powerhouse, so congrats on making it this far! Prepare to increase your Pilates game in this part as we ratchet it up with a number of energizing movements. We will concentrate on pushing your body with dynamic routines that will improve your balance, strength, and flexibility. As you go through these workouts, you'll be pushing yourself to new heights with the help of step-by-step directions and professional advice. In order to crush these Wall Pilates Workouts like never before, let's lace up our Pilates shoes.

WALL SQUATS WITH LEG LIFTS

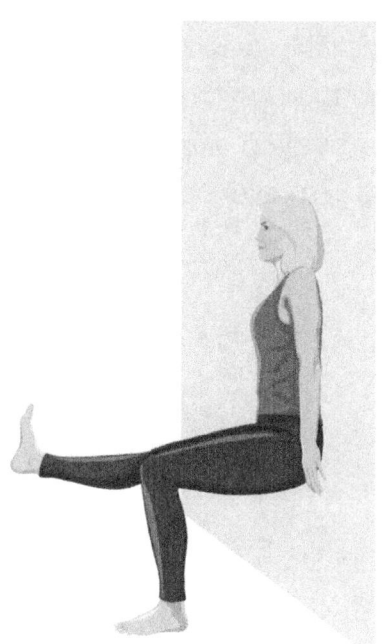

1.

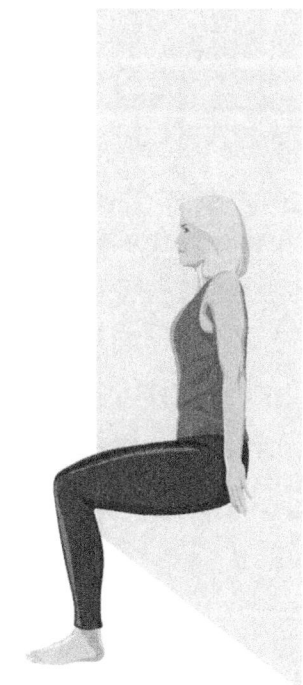

2.

This exercise works your core muscles as well as the muscles in your legs, especially the quadriceps and glutes.

INSTRUCTIONS:

1. Place your feet shoulder-width apart and stand with your back to the wall. Your knees should be 90 degrees bent and your thighs should be parallel to the floor as you descend the wall.
2. Raise your arms straight in front of you or place your hands on your hips.
3. Slowly lift one leg up to 90 degrees, then lower it back down and repeat
4. Perform 10 to 15 repetitions on each side, or for a predetermined period of time.

- Ensure that your knees do not extend past your toes and are directly above your ankles.
- Throughout the entire movement, maintain a tight core and a straight back.
- As you lift and drop your leg, pay attention to maintaining your body's stability against the wall.

WALL SITS

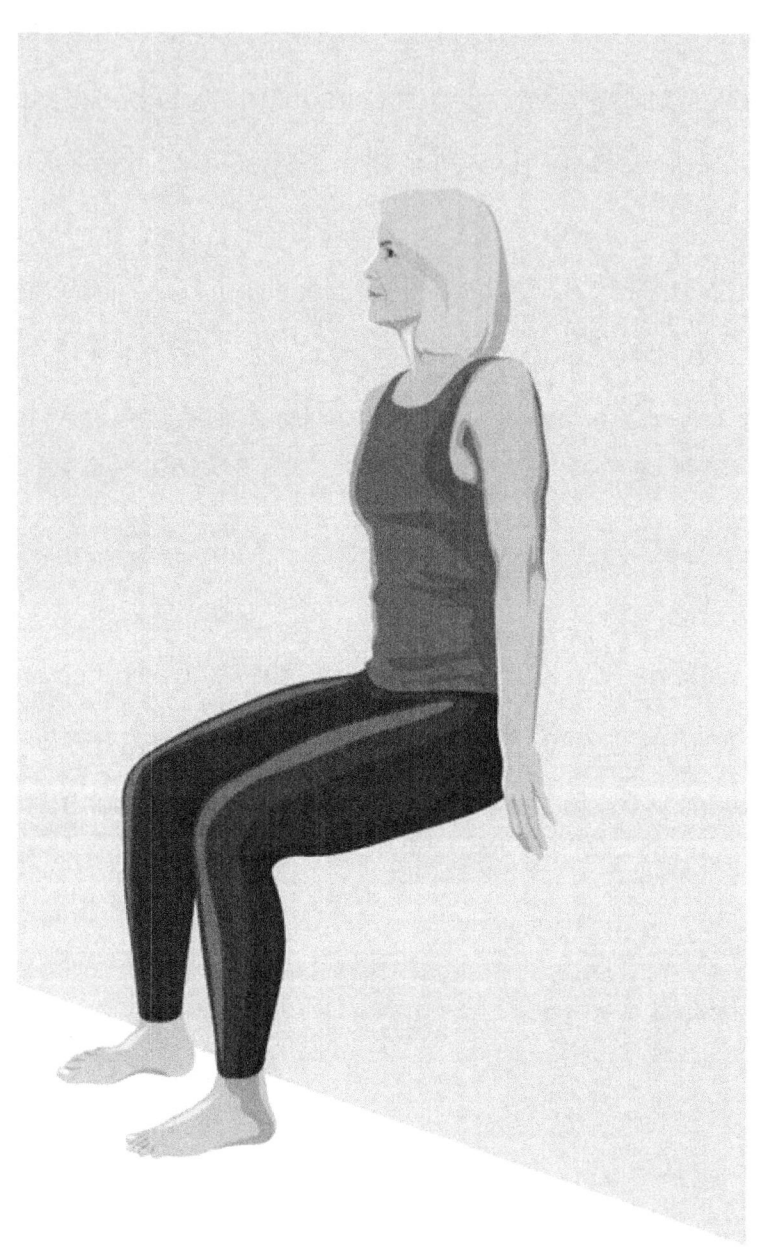

The exercise known as the wall sit tones and strengthens the muscles in the legs and glutes. Additionally, this workout can increase lower body strength and endurance.

INSTRUCTIONS:

1. Place your feet shoulder-width apart and stand with your back to the wall. Your knees should be 90 degrees bent and your thighs should be parallel to the floor as you descend the wall.
2. Contract the muscles in your core and maintain a straight back. As long as you are able to, up to a minute, maintain this posture.
3. After taking a few deep breaths, slowly stand back up to your starting posture. Repeat this motion many times.

- Ensure that your knees do not extend past your toes and are directly above your ankles.
- Throughout the entire movement, maintain a tight core and a straight back.
- Holding a medicine ball or weights in your hands will make the exercise harder.

WALL ROLL-DOWNS

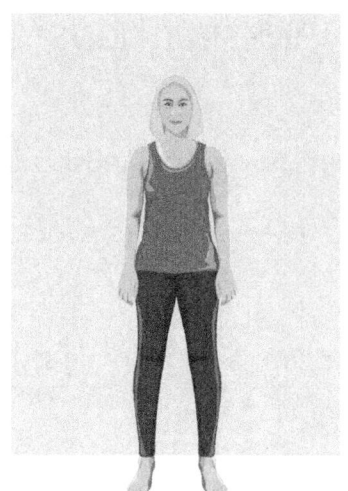

1.

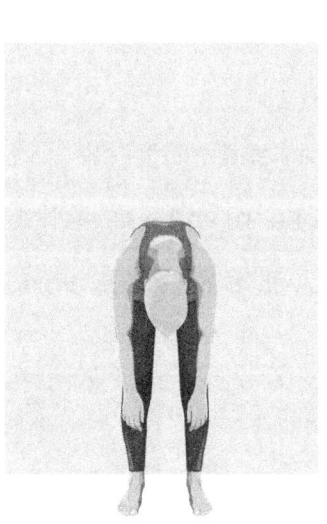

2.

3.

Pilates exercises like wall rolls down aim to stretch and strengthen your spine, enhance posture, and ease neck and shoulder tension. Your body is supported throughout this exercise by a wall.

INSTRUCTIONS:

1. Place your hands on the wall at shoulder height while standing facing the wall with your feet hip-distance apart.
2. Take a big breath in, then, as you exhale, start to roll your spine down toward the floor while keeping your feet firmly planted.
3. Roll down as far as you can while maintaining a relaxed head and neck that are parallel to your spine.
4. After pausing and inhaling deeply at the bottom of the movement, carefully roll one vertebra at a time back up to the beginning position.
5. Continue doing this multiple times, moving each time gently and fluidly.

- Start slowly and concentrate on appropriate form: It's crucial to start slowly and concentrate on proper form when completing Wall Roll-Downs. You'll be able to avoid harm and benefit the most from the exercise if you do this.
- Breathe in and out to assist you progress through the workout easily.
- As you start to tumble down the wall, take a deep breath in and let it out.
- Be careful to maintain relaxed shoulders as you roll down the wall. By doing so, you'll be able to reduce shoulder and neck stress and improve the stretch in your spine.

WALL MOUNTAIN CLIMBERS

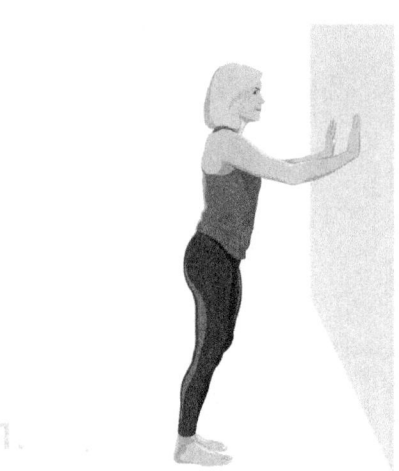

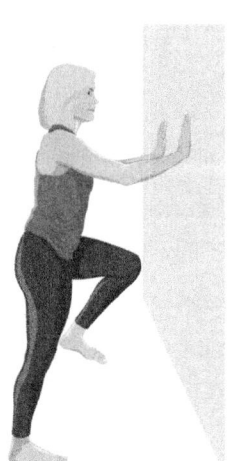

Exercises like Wall Mountain Climbers, which work your core, upper body, and legs, are dynamic and difficult. This exercise simulates the motion of ascending a mountain and works several muscle groups while giving the heart a terrific cardiovascular workout.

INSTRUCTIONS:

1. Start by assuming a high plank posture with your back to the wall, your hands exactly beneath your shoulders, and your feet up against the wall.
2. Maintain a straight line from your head to your heels by engaging your core.
3. Alternately bring one knee to your chest while extending the other leg behind you while keeping your upper body steady.
4. Change legs quickly, bringing the bent leg back and the extended leg forward.
5. As though you were scaling a mountain, keep your breathing controlled and your movement steady.
6. Continue alternating legs for a desired number of repetitions or a specific duration.

- To balance your body and keep appropriate form throughout the exercise, concentrate on keeping your core engaged.
- Maintain a relaxed neck and keep your shoulders away from your ears.
- To avoid hip slumping or raising too high, maintain a firm plank stance.

WALL LEG SWINGS

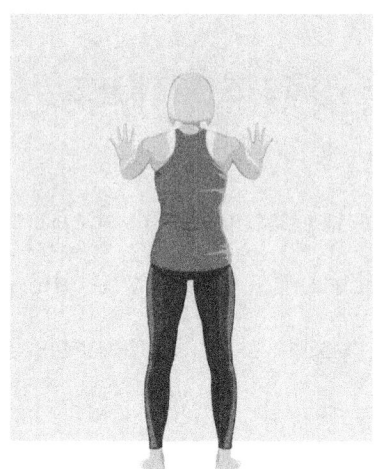

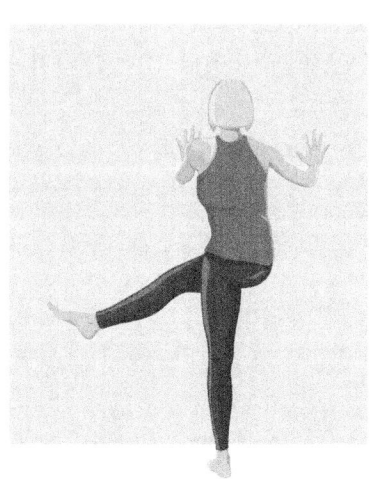

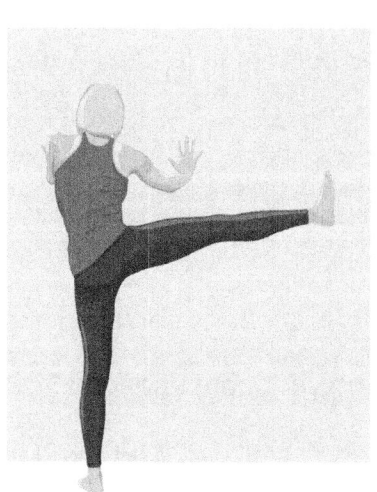

Leg swings against the wall are an excellent way to increase hip and leg flexibility and mobility. It's also advised to warm up the lower body before exercising.

INSTRUCTIONS:

1. To start, turn to the side with your arms outstretched and place your hands at shoulder height against the wall.
2. Stand with your feet hip-width apart to keep your weight evenly distributed.
3. Maintain a straight spine and use your abdominal muscles.
4. Swing your right leg slowly forward and backward against the wall while keeping it straight.
5. Swing your right leg ten to twelve times, then repeat with your left.
6. After completing the set, take a little pause before performing two more sets.

- Start with little swings and build up to bigger swings to get accustomed to the exercise.
- As you exercise, contract your abdominal muscles to maintain a straight back.
- Avoiding abrupt leg swings will benefit your hips and lower back.
- Keep your focus on fully exhaling as you swing your leg forward.

DAYS 26-28

Welcome to the last days of the Wall Pilates Workouts. Congratulations on completing the challenge's final phase! You are nearly there! I have some carefully chosen exercises in this final section to assist you finish the course successfully. Your body and mind will continue to be challenged by these exercises . Let's get started and finish strong, knowing that you have a few days left to complete this amazing voyage. Keep up the fantastic effort and finish on a high note!

WALL ANGELS

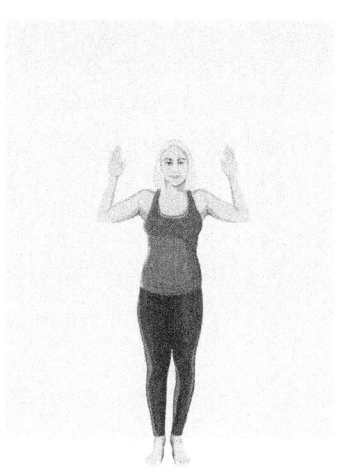

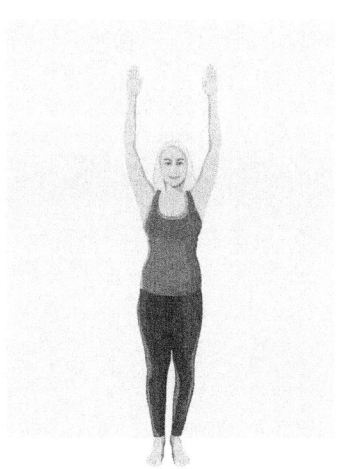
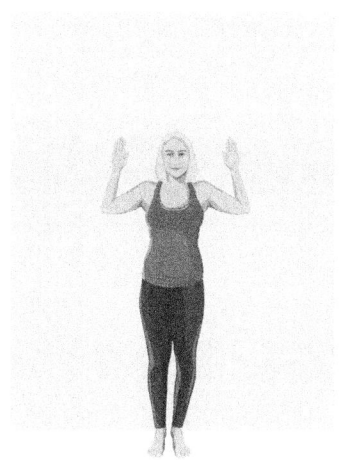

The upper back and shoulders' muscles are toned and strengthened with the wall angel workout. Additionally, this exercise can help with posture and spinal alignment.

INSTRUCTIONS:

1. Stand with your back to the wall and your feet shoulder-width apart. Keep your shoulders relaxed while contracting your abdominal muscles.
2. Bring your hands up to the level of your ears while raising your arms to shoulder height and bending your elbows.
3. Slowly slide your arms up the wall, keeping your elbows bent and your hands close to your ears. Make sure your shoulders stay relaxed and your back stays flat against the wall.
4. Hold this position for a few breaths, then slowly lower your arms back down to the starting position.
5. Repeat for several repetitions, focusing on maintaining proper form throughout the entire movement.

- Keep your shoulders relaxed and away from your ears.
- If you find it challenging to keep your hands close to your ears, try using a small towel or resistance band to keep your elbows in place.
- Focus on breathing deeply and evenly throughout the exercise.

WALL LEG CIRCLES

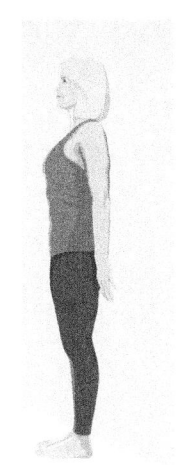

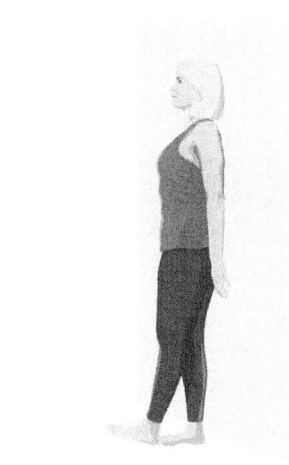
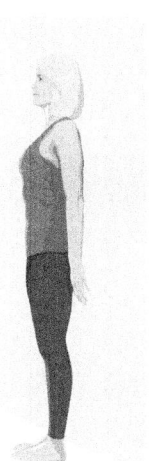

Wall Leg Circles involves moving the legs in circles while maintaining a straight back, which engages the core and enhances stability.

INSTRUCTIONS:

1. Start by standing upright, with your back against the wall and feet hips-width apart
2. Slightly lift your right leg up
3. Draw small circles with your foot

TIP:

- To maintain stability and safeguard your lower back, keep your core tight and your lower back pressed firmly against the wall throughout he exercise.
- As your strength and flexibility improve, start with small circles and progressively enlarge them.
- Pay attention to maintaining smooth, controlled motions and avoiding any jerky or unexpected ones.

WALL TEASERS

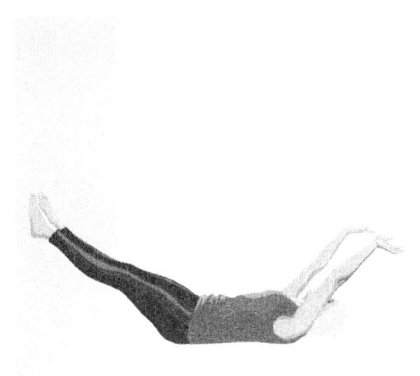

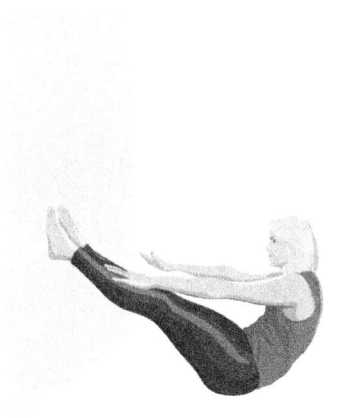
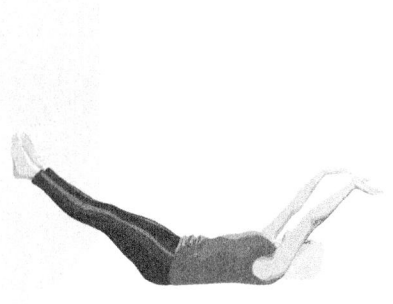

The Wall Teasers works the lower back, obliques, and other core muscles. It calls for balance and control, making it a useful exercise for building core strength and enhancing stability.

INSTRUCTIONS:

1. Stretch your legs while resting on the floor with your knees bent and your feet up against a wall.
2. Start by raising your arms over your head. Next, engage your core muscles by moving your belly button toward your legs while keeping a straight posture.
3. Your feet should remain on the wall as you roll back down.
4. Return your spine to the floor with control as you slowly reverse the action by lowering your upper body and legs to the beginning position.

- As you elevate your core, tense your abs and obliques to prevent your lower back from arching or rounding.
- If you find it difficult to maintain your legs straight, you can bend your knees slightly or use a strap over your feet to help with the movement.
- Start with smaller motions and progressively expand the range of motion as you build strength and stability.

CONCLUSION

As we reach the end of this 28-day challenge guide for wall pilates workouts, I hope you've seen how this practice can help you in many ways. Over the past four weeks, you've learned how to use the wall to improve your flexibility, balance, and posture, and you've been introduced to a variety of exercises that will help you reach your goals.

I want to stress how important it is to practice often, pay attention to your body, and be patient with yourself. Wall pilates is not a quick fix, but rather a way of life that you have to commit to and keep up with. But I'm sure you've already started to see the benefits of wall pilates and know that the work is well worth it.

Remember that wall pilates can help you in more ways than just your body. As you do the exercises, you will also feel calmer and more relaxed, and you will find new ways to connect with your body. This can be a powerful way to deal with stress and worry and feel better about yourself in general.

I think you should keep doing wall pilates after this 28-day challenge is over. Set yourself new goals and keep giving yourself new tasks to push yourself. Join a class in your area or work out with a friend to keep yourself inspired and answerable. The journey doesn't end here; there's always more to learn and find out about your body.

Lastly, I want to thank you for picking this guide and deciding to use wall pilates to improve your health and well-being. I hope that this guide has been helpful, interesting, and motivating for you, and that you will keep looking into the many benefits of wall pilates for years to come.

You got this!
Lisa

Printed in Great Britain
by Amazon